“THE BAKER ACT”

WRITTEN BY: CAMERON R. MITCHELL JR

Illustrated by: Sketco Studio

Disclaimer

This book and all of its contents are a work of fiction. All of the names, characters, places, events, incidents, and locations are a product of the author's imagination and are intended to be used in a fictitious manner.

Any resemblance to any person, living or dead, or the events of the story is purely coincidental.
The author cannot be held responsible for any personal or commercial damage arising from communication, application, or misinterpretation of the information presented herein.

Contents

Author's Introduction

This storyline seeks to promote compassion, empathy, and awareness of mental health struggles. It sheds light on the damaging effects of bullying and unprofessional behavior—particularly in settings where individuals seek healing and support. The narrative also reveals the absence of kindness in such environments, emphasizing how this lack can deepen a patient's suffering. At its heart, the story explores the transformative power of love and kindness as divine gifts, embodied by an anointed healer whose appearance invites skepticism.

Despite facing doubt and prejudice, this healer becomes a vessel of hope and change, challenging assumptions and inspiring grace.

Baker Act: Brief History Overview

The Baker Act, formally known as the Florida Mental Health Act of 1971, allows designated professionals—such as physicians, licensed mental health practitioners, judges, and law enforcement officers—to initiate an involuntary mental health examination for individuals experiencing a psychiatric crisis. Named after State Representative Maxine Baker, a strong advocate for mental health reform, the Act aims to provide timely and appropriate care in a secure environment while protecting individual rights.

To qualify for involuntary examination, a person must be believed to have a mental illness and, as a result, pose a danger to themselves or others, or be unable to care for themselves. The individual can be held for up to 72 hours in a designated receiving facility for evaluation and stabilization. During this period, licensed professionals assess whether the person meets the criteria for further involuntary treatment or if alternative services are more appropriate. After the 72-hour window, the individual may be released, agree to voluntary treatment, or face a court petition for continued involuntary care.

The core goals of the Baker Act are to ensure immediate stabilization, safeguard individual rights, and determine the most suitable path for ongoing treatment and recovery.

The Baker Act

Travis, a 28-year-old young adult, was placed under the Baker Act by the police after being caught staring at the sky for long periods of time, as some civilians claimed he might be a threat to himself. He was sent to a dark, creepy hospital and diagnosed with schizophrenia. The psychologist informed him of his diagnosis. Travis seemed confused by the results, and the doctor believed he might be delusional and overwhelmed by his strong faith in God. Travis experienced tingling sensations and sweating in the palms of his hands, but he is uncertain about why this seems to occur and is trying to figure out a deeper meaning behind it.

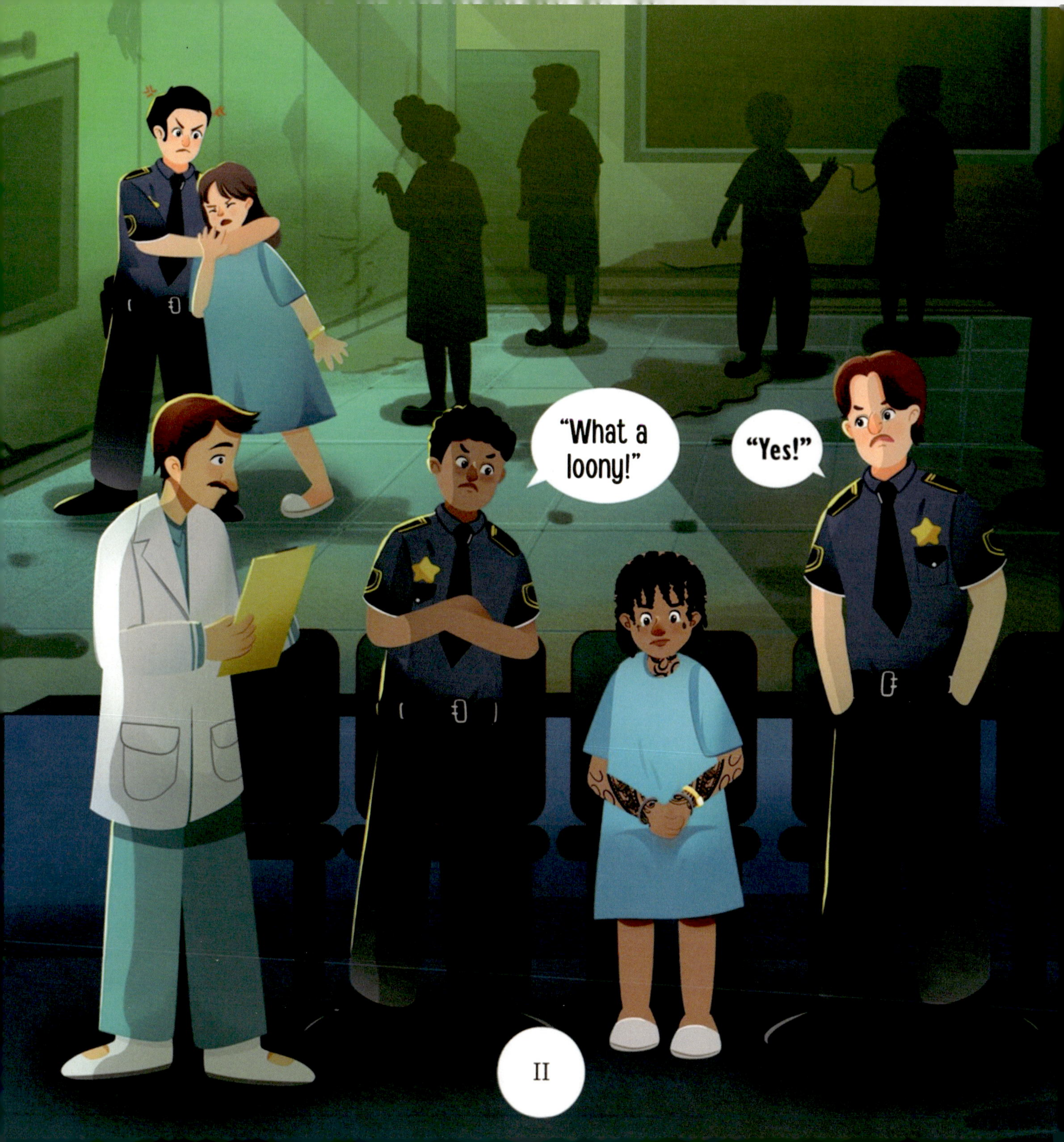
"What a loony!"
"Yes!"

Travis finds himself not really having anyone to talk to during lunchtime on the behavior unit floor where he was placed. He is being mistreated and stereotyped by nurses because of the tattoos on his face and the gold teeth that seems unsuitable for a young man. Other patients on the floor seem terrified and disgusted of him because of his outward appearance.

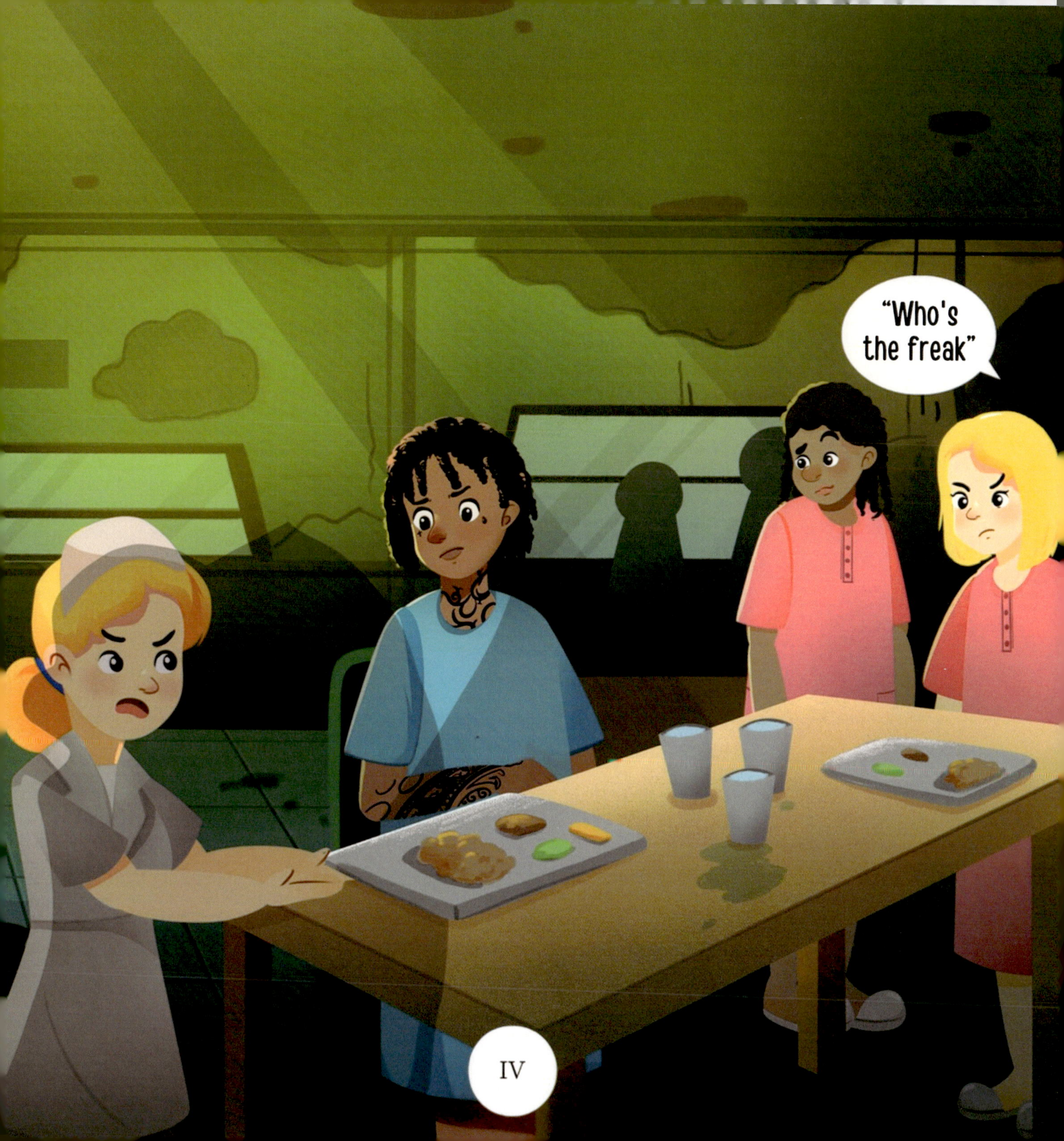
"Who's the freak"

On a Tuesday morning, Travis encounters a scenario in the hallway of the behavioral unit, where he observes another patient being subjected to ridicule due to her stumbling and stuttering, symptoms that appear to be caused by the medication administered by the medical staff. This individual grapples with low self-esteem, prompting her to engage in self-harm as a means of alleviating her emotional pain. Rather than confronting the aggressive patient, Travis chooses to approach both individuals with compassion.
He reassures the young woman, Brittany, that her beauty cannot be defined by others; rather, she must recognize it within herself without seeking external validation. He emphasizes that self-harm will not rectify her low self-esteem; only a shift in her mindset can foster true healing from within.

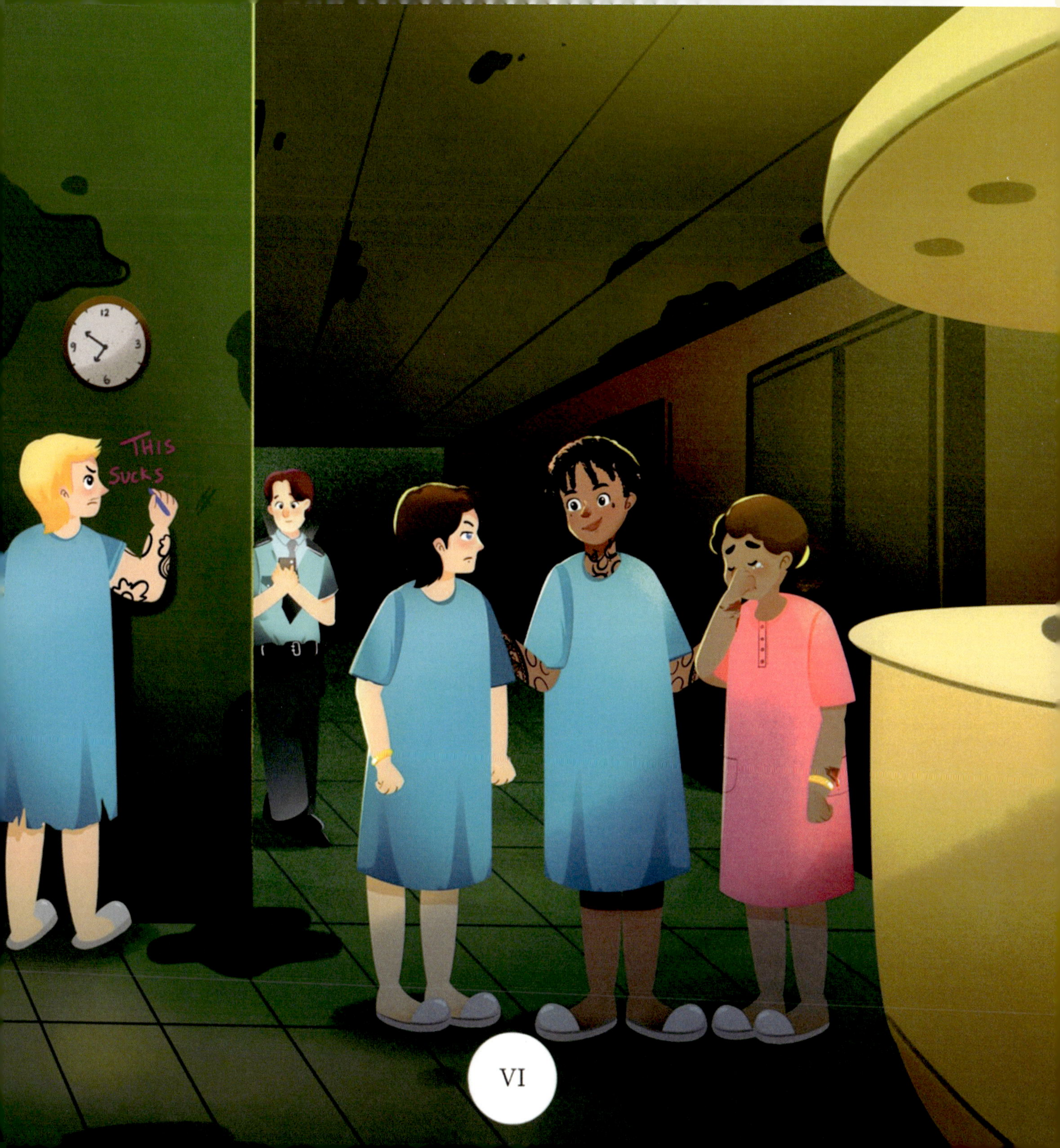
THIS SUCKS

In that moment, Travis feels the sweat on his hands and senses something deeper—a spiritual gift stirring within him. While comforting John, a patient battling drug addiction and abandonment, Travis speaks words of hope and love. As he encourages him, John experiences a sudden lift in his spirit and a change in his body, as if something unseen begins to heal him. Travis tells John he is important, chosen to do great things, and deeply loved by God. It's then that Travis begins to understand his calling: to be a vessel of healing, encouragement, and faith—doing God's work through compassion and grace.

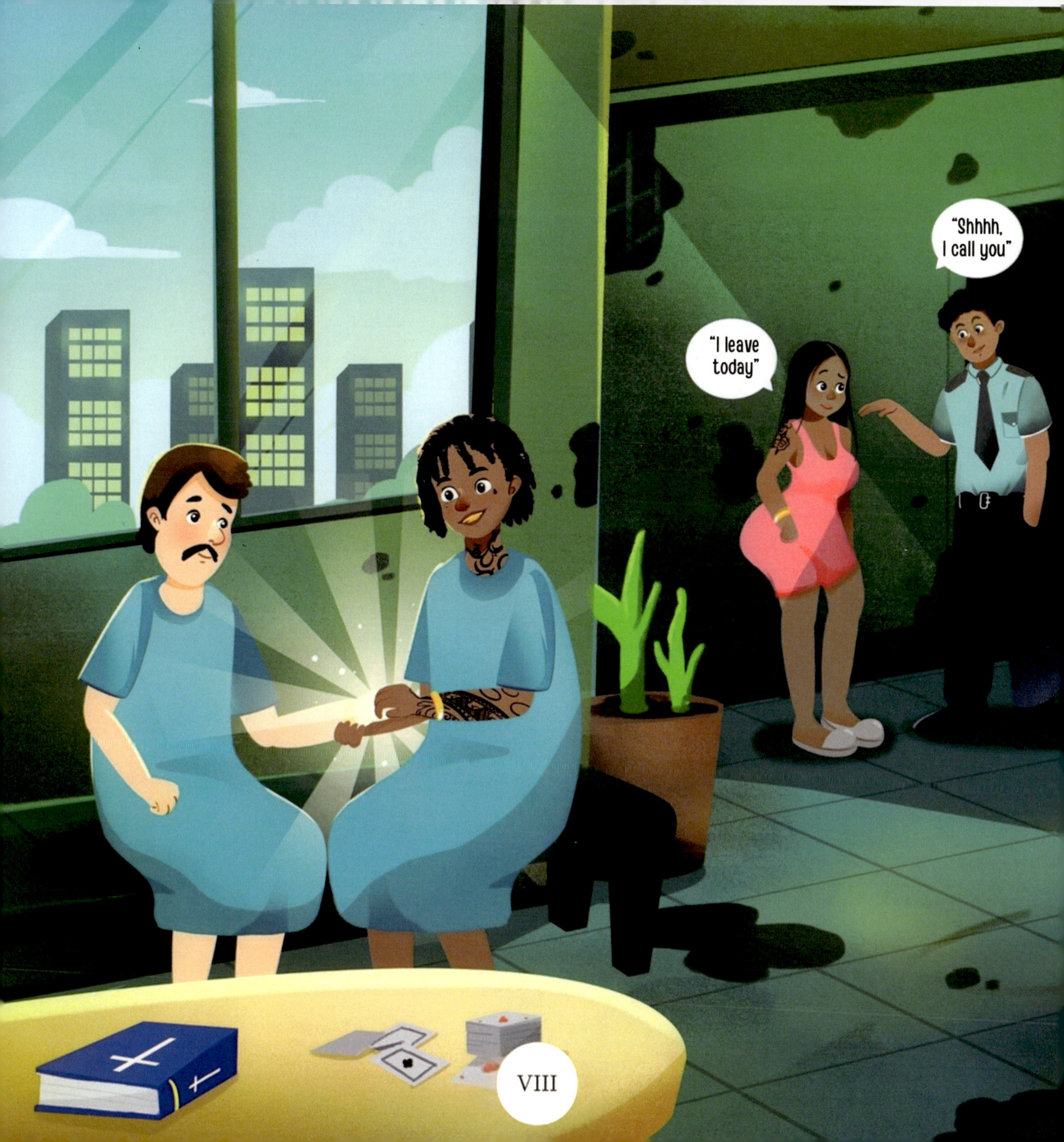
"I leave today"
"Shhhh, I call you"

The doctors and staff dismissed Travis with cold skepticism, brushing off his gift as mere fantasy. It unsettled them that patients sought his presence more than their prescriptions, drawn to the quiet strength and peace he carried. His healing didn't follow protocol—it followed purpose. To them, that made him a threat. But Travis never argued. He simply kept showing up, letting the power within him speak where words were no longer needed.

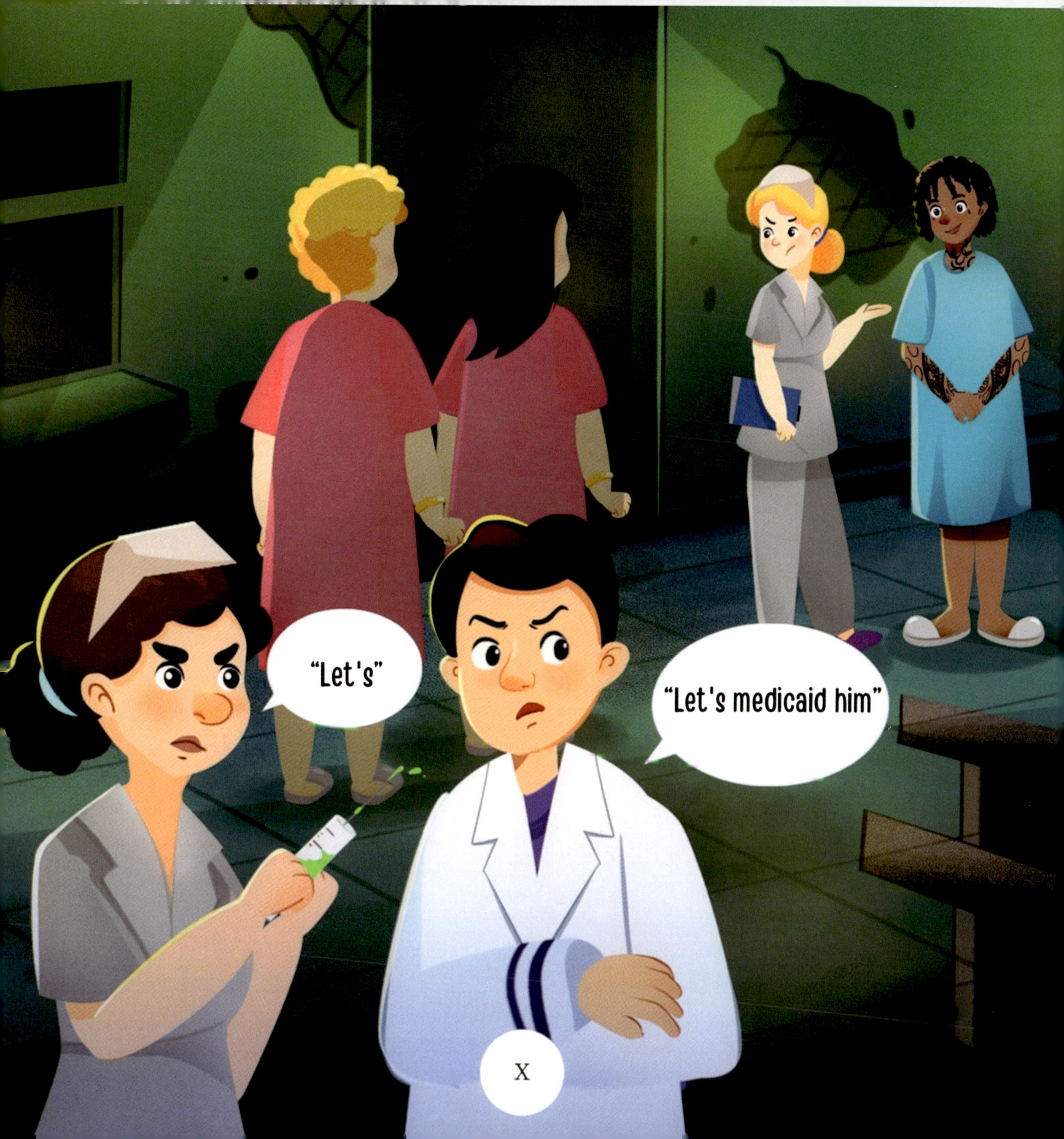
"Let's"
"Let's medicaid him"

Despite the staff's opposition and evident disdain, Travis remains steadfast in his commitment to employ his God-given gift in healing others, faithfully upholding his divine calling to serve God's people.

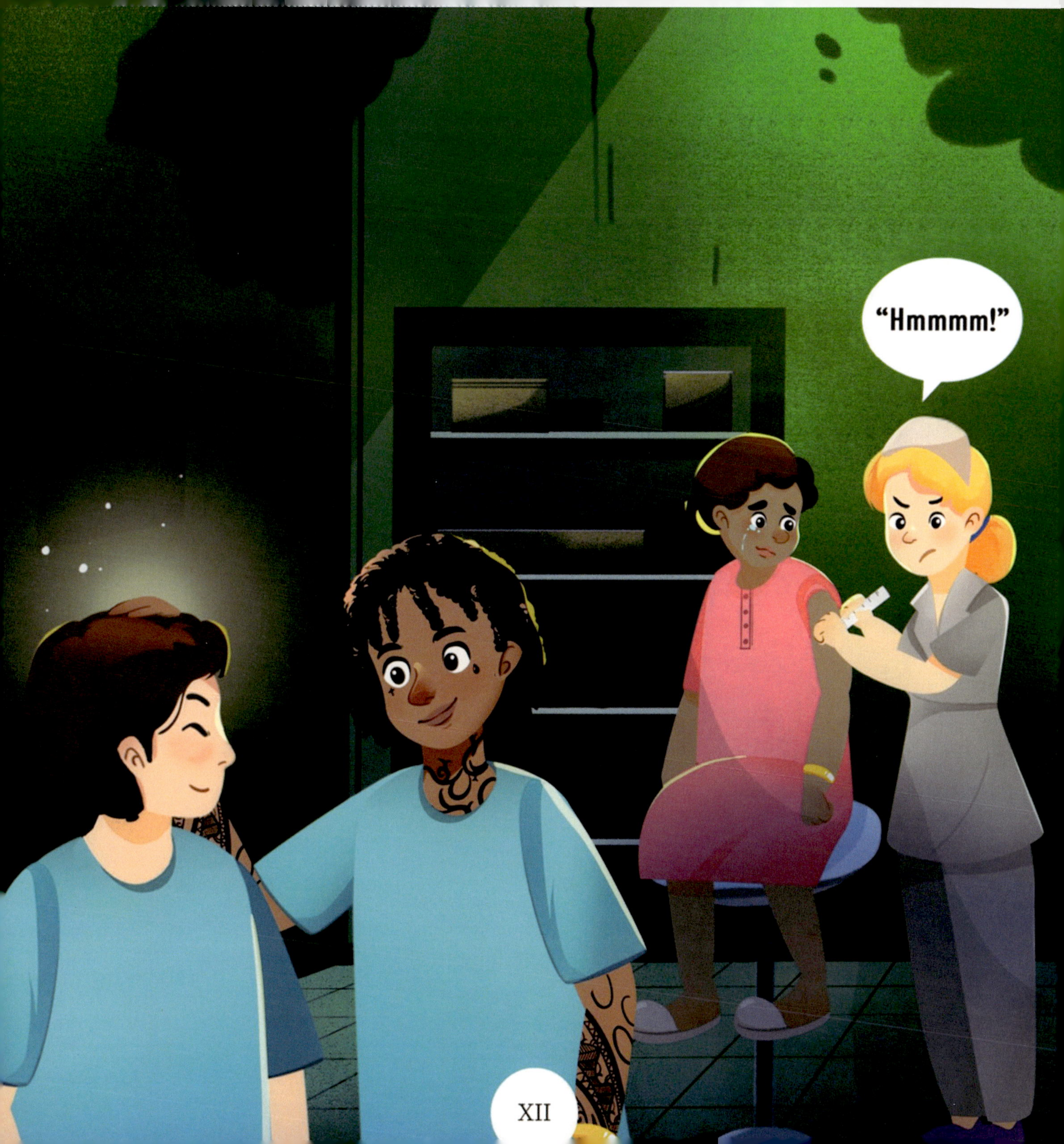
"Hmmmm!"

The staff begins to observe the positive transformations in the patients whom Travis has prayed—transformations that no medication could effect. Despite Mark's initial aggressive behavior towards the medical staff and his refusal to adhere to his prescribed medication, he has demonstrated remarkable humility and sincerity as a result of the encouragement and healing provided by Travis. Consequently, Mark has evolved into a person greater than what others had anticipated.

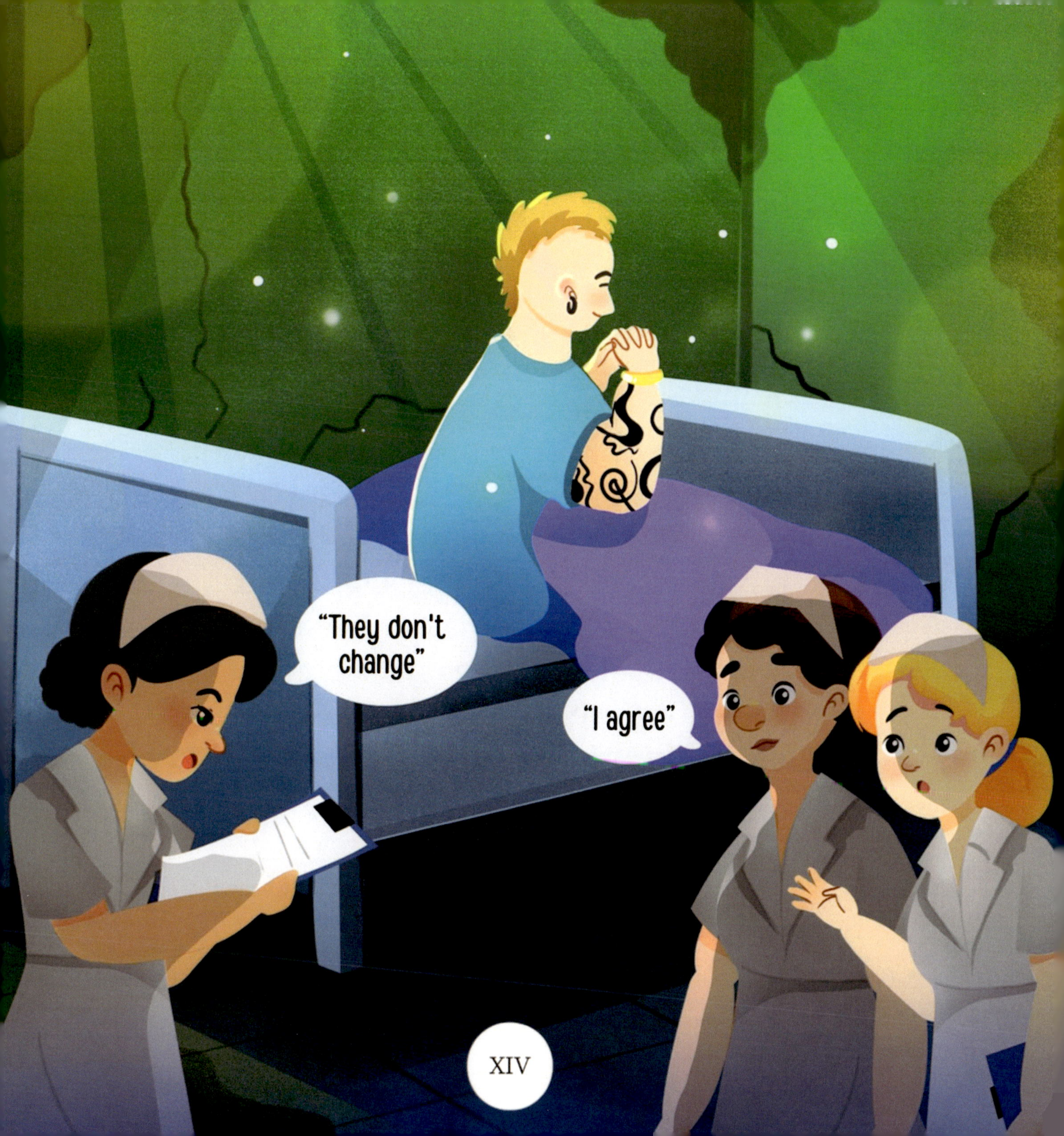
"They don't change"
"I agree"

The doctors and staff begin to examine Travis's gift in search of a scientific explanation—yet, like many in the scientific community, they are hindered by a lack of understanding rooted in disbelief. Though a patient within their facility, Travis refuses to let his circumstances—or their theories—diminish his sense of purpose or make him feel inferior. He remains confident in the divine origin of his gift.

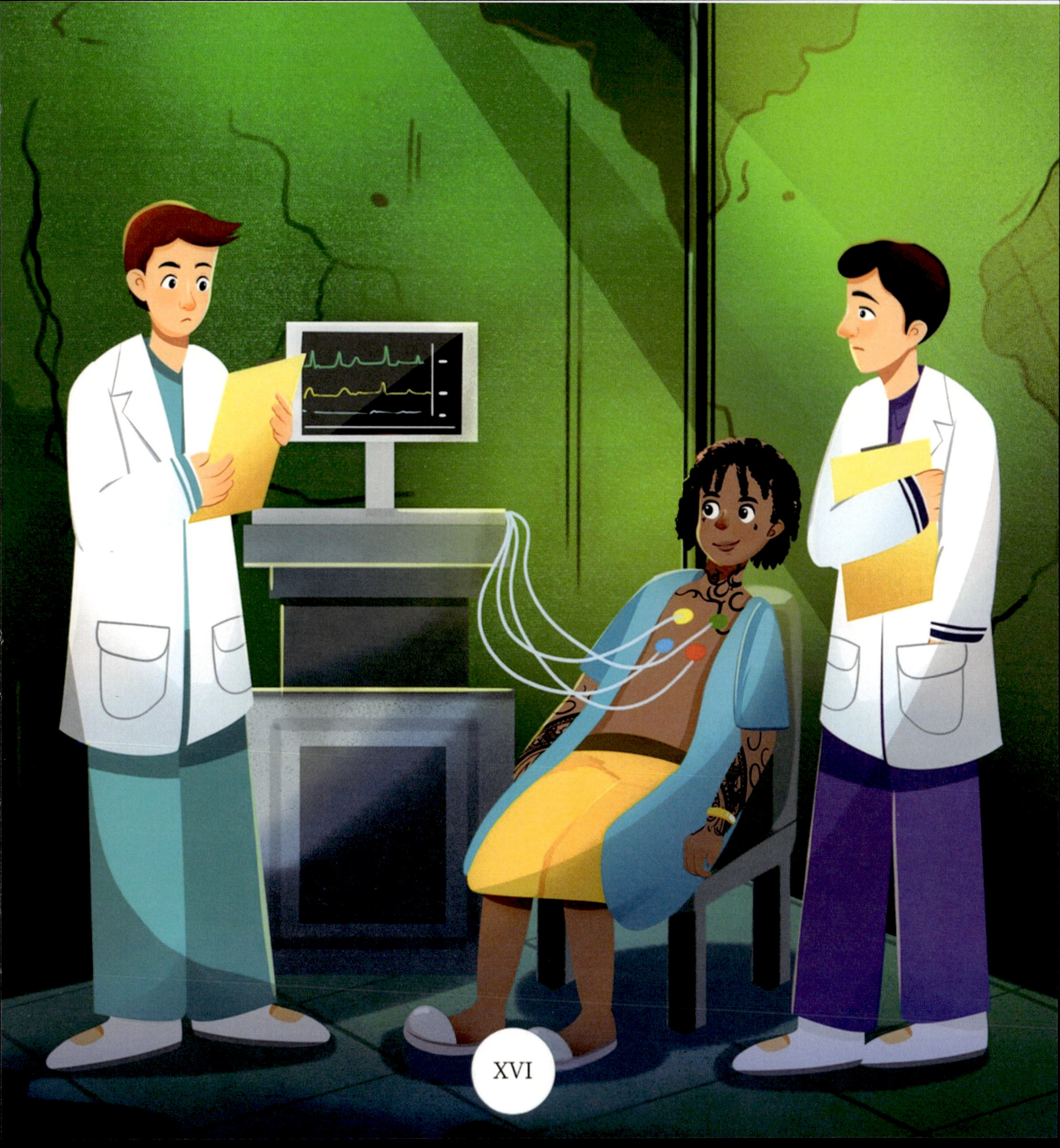

Travis's gift is ultimately revealed to be a genuine spiritual phenomenon—one that transcends scientific explanation. During a moment of observation, Dr. Rothstein witnesses Travis begin to tremble in his hospital bed. As Rothstein touches his arm, he is suddenly drawn into a vivid vision—transported into Travis's childhood, a realm of memory and trauma known only to Travis himself. In this powerful moment, Rothstein experiences firsthand the emotional weight and pain that shaped Travis's life. Upon awakening, Travis calmly tells him, 'You can bury your trauma now.' It is then that Rothstein understands, perhaps for the first time, why he became a psychiatrist—not merely to heal others, but to confront and heal his own wounds. This encounter marks a new beginning for both men, serving as a profound reminder to approach others with humility and compassion—for they may carry extraordinary gifts that defy human understanding.

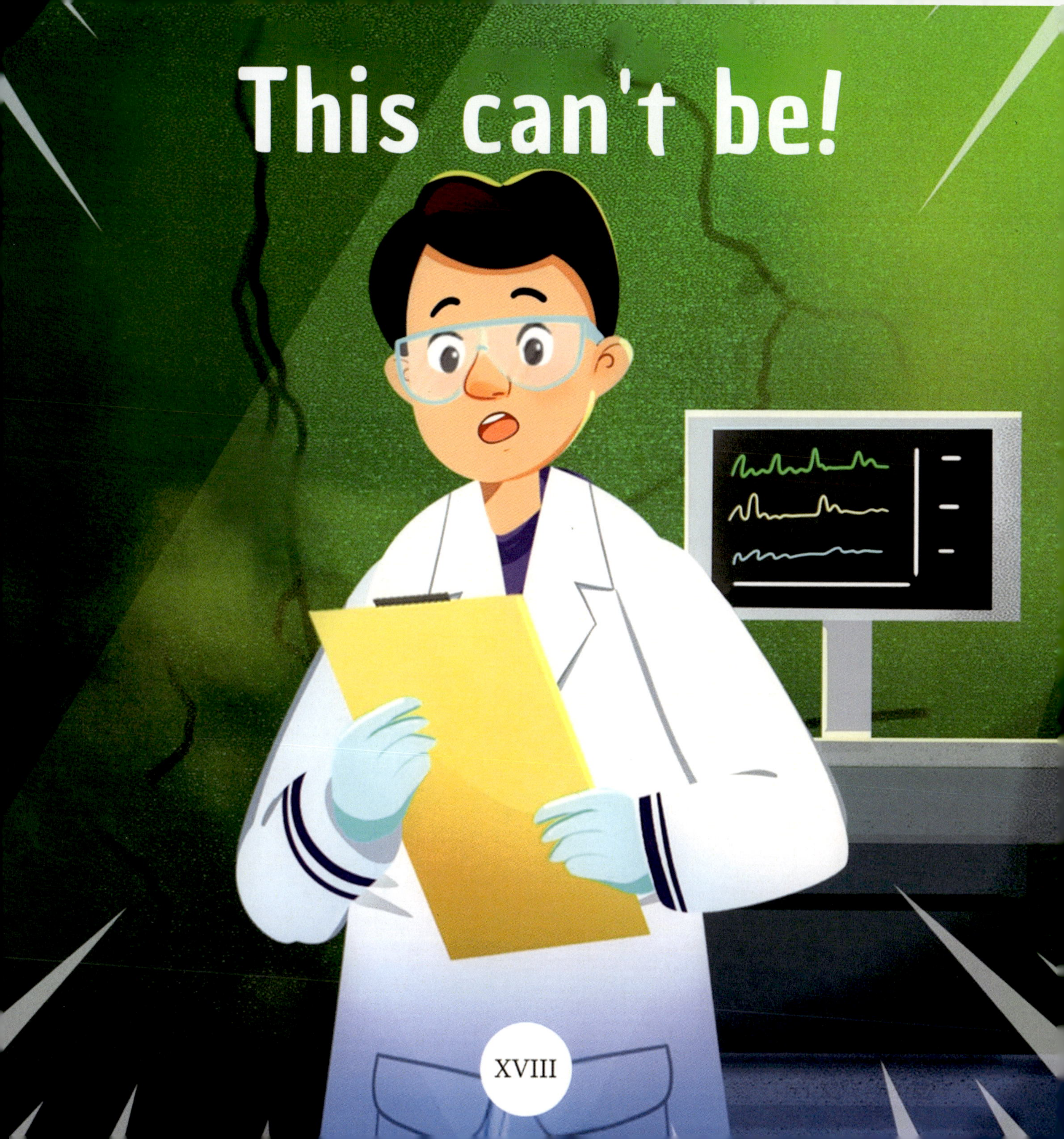
This can't be!

The staff, once dismissive, grows quiet in the light of Travis's presence. With time, they begin to treat him with kindness—not out of pity, but reverence. Something in him speaks without words, a calling too profound to ignore.

He shines—not with pride, but with purpose. And in that quiet radiance, even the most openhearted are moved to tears. They see not just a man, but a soul on fire with meaning.

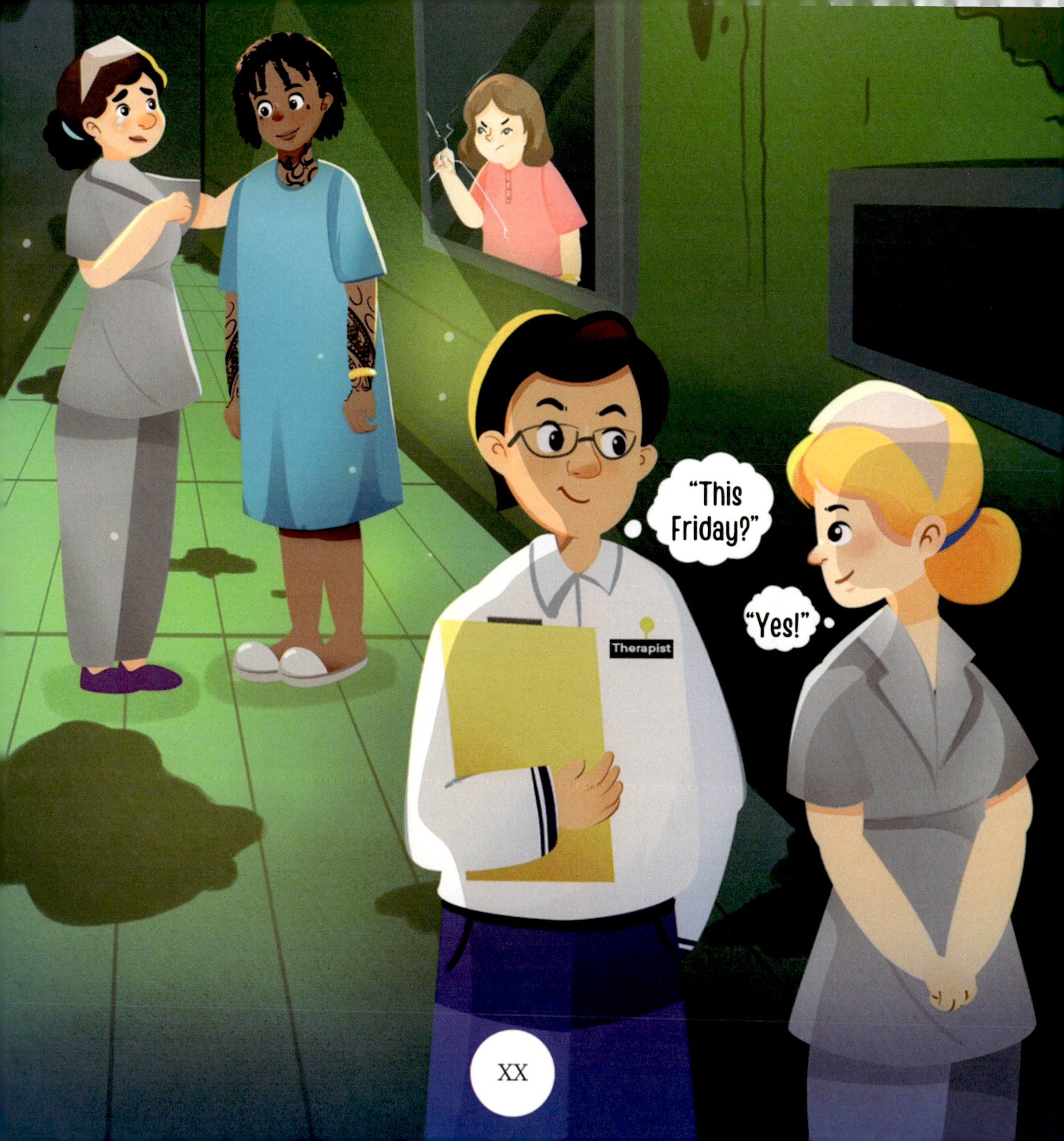
"This Friday?"
"Yes!"
Therapist

Travis's quiet gift of healing stirs something in the hearts of the staff. Watching him, they begin to reevaluate everything they thought they knew about care. His presence reveals a deeper medicine—one not found in bottles or charts, but in compassion, stillness, and connection.

They come to see that healing isn't always about curing. Sometimes, it's about listening. Sometimes, it's about simply being. And in that space, they realize: not every wound needs a pill—some just need a touch of grace.

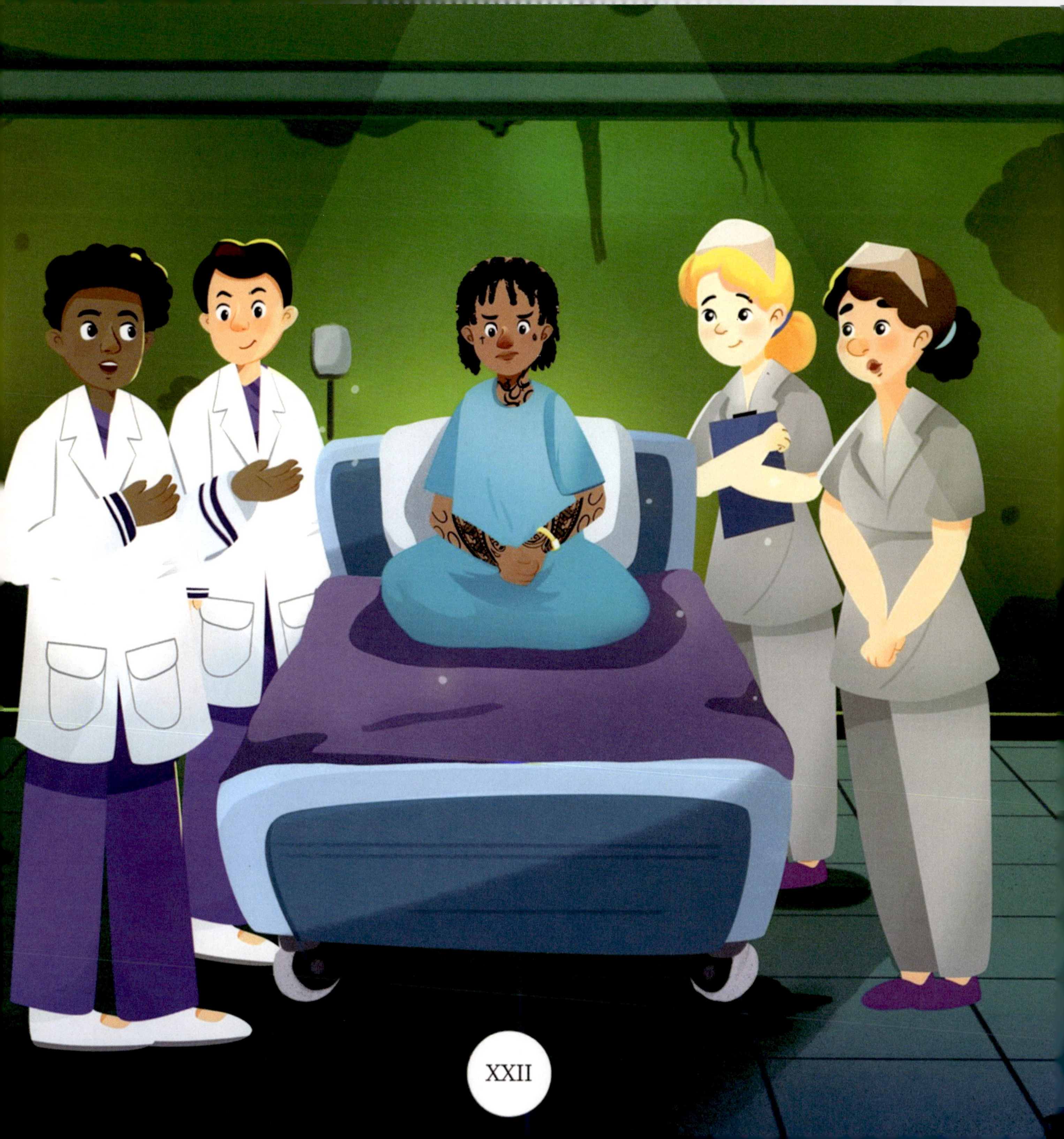

Under Travis's guidance, the hospital has become more than a place of healing—it has become a sanctuary of compassion and love. His influence has reshaped the atmosphere, infusing the halls with grace, empathy, and quiet strength. The staff, inspired by his example, approach each patient with renewed purpose—swift to hear, slow to speak, and always ready to serve with open hearts.

Through his leadership, care is no longer just clinical—it is personal, prayerful, and profound. His presence doesn't just guide—it transforms, reminding everyone around him that healing begins not only with medicine, but with mercy, kindness, and the love of God at work through human hands.

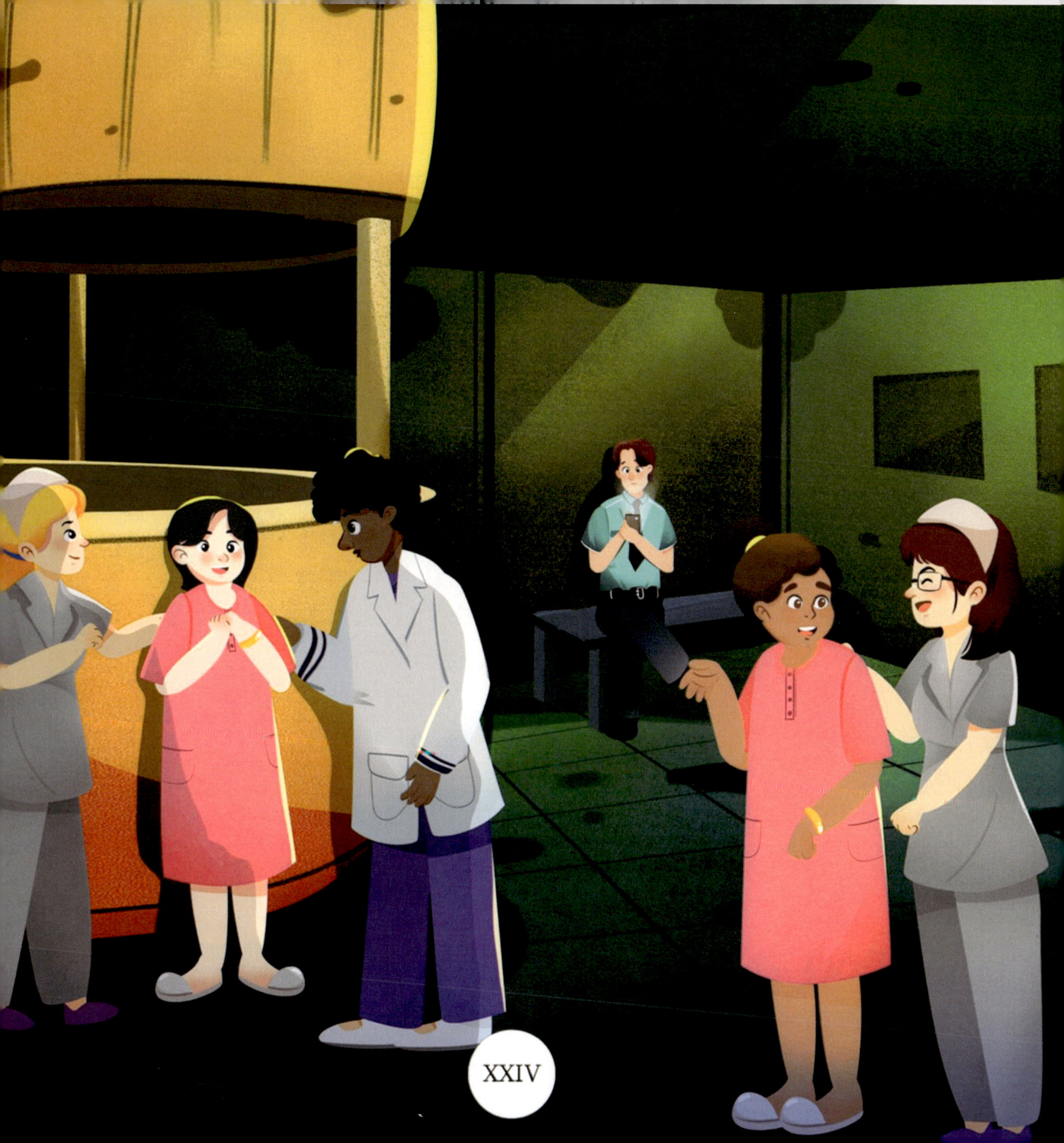

Travis's story and his deep compassion for others inspire hearts to awaken, faith to deepen, and lives to change. Through his example, people are drawn closer to God, moved to serve, and empowered to lead with the same grace and purpose that he so faithfully embodies.

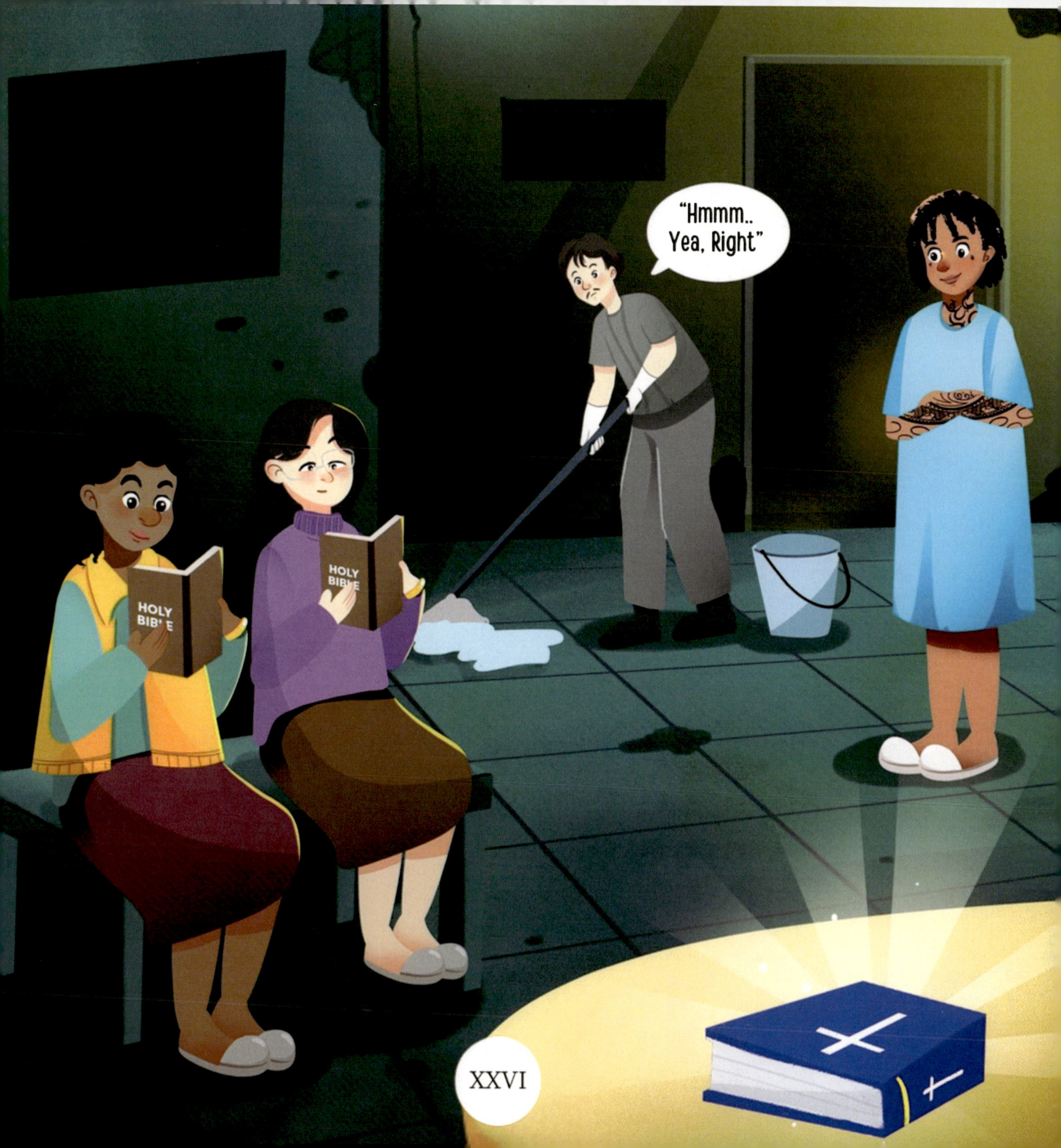
"Hmmm..
Yea, Right"
HOLY BIBLE
HOLY BIBLE

The medical team is astonished to witness Tina and Rebecca—both with histories of abuse by men and considered at high risk for suicide—openly embrace Travis, showing trust and gradually sharing their thoughts with him. His approach is different: gentle, patient, and free of judgment. He listens without trying to fix, and speaks with quiet empathy rather than authority.

Through his steady presence and compassionate words, Travis helps them see themselves not as victims, but as survivors. He reminds them that pain, though cruel and undeserved, can be a path to strength. His words resonate: sometimes we must endure suffering to grow beyond the limits others—or life—have placed on us. In their most painful moments, Tina and Rebecca begin to rediscover who they truly are and what they're capable of becoming.

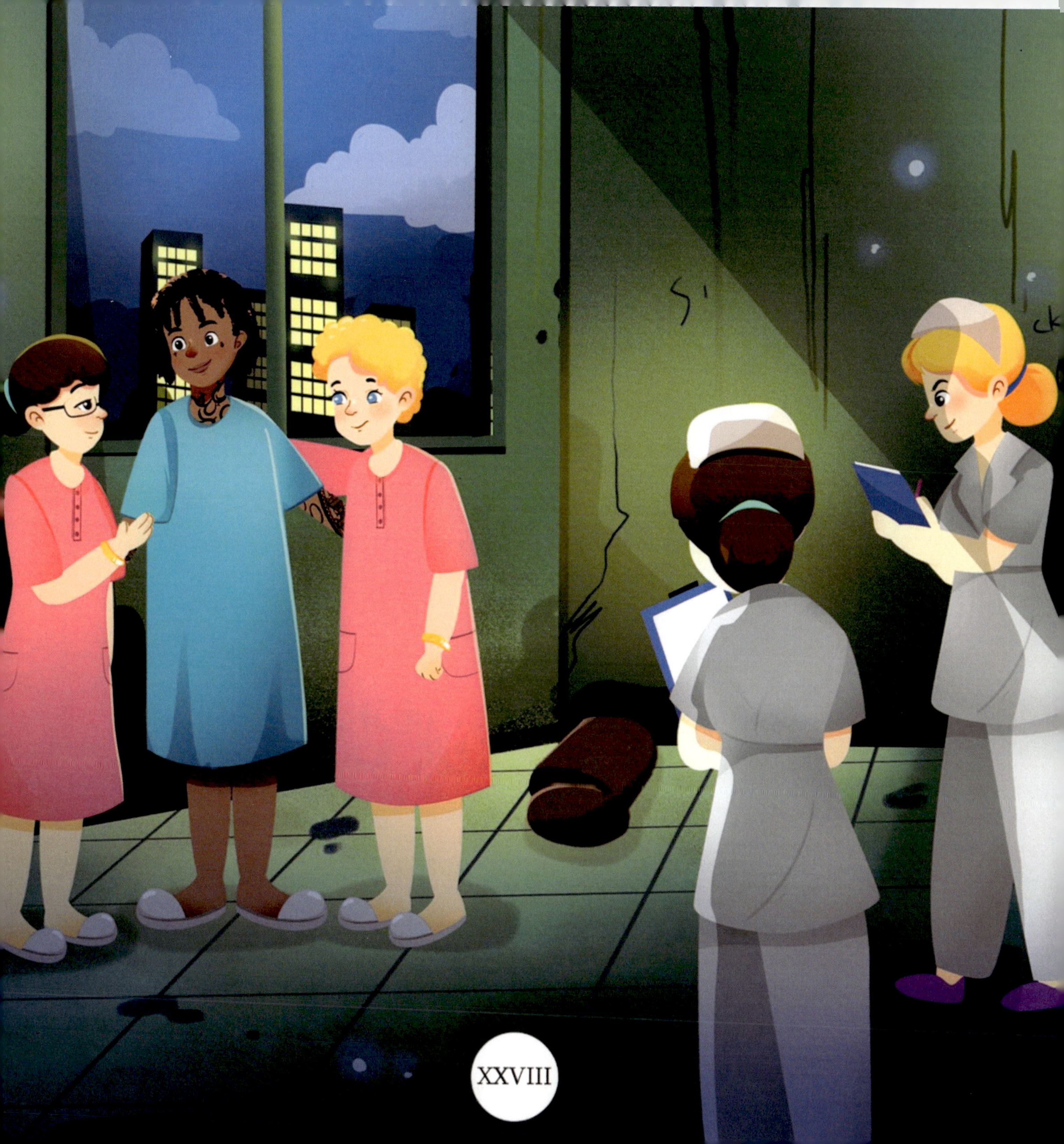

Travis is healing, inspiring, and igniting hearts with every touch. His gift is a divine spark—a holy fire fueled by the boundless love and compassion God has woven into our very being. The sweat of his hands is no ordinary labor; it is a powerful prayer in motion, a sacred offering that lights the darkness and reminds us that even through pain, beauty can rise—and through faith, miracles unfold.

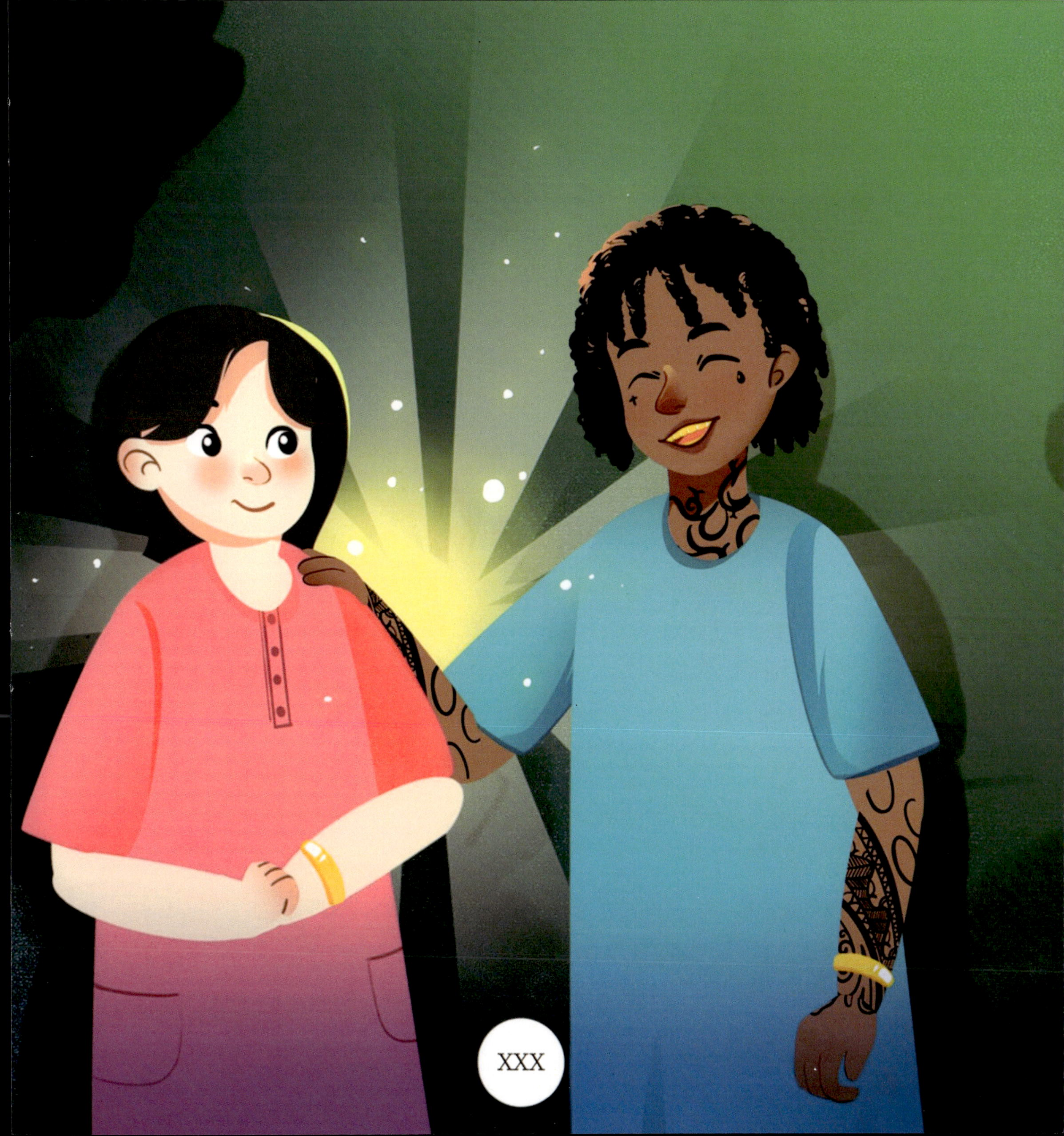

The hospital has become a model for compassionate care, due to Travis's influence. It is now a place of fellowship where patients are pleased to witness the positive changes—a new beginning where both treatment and voluntary support offer them a welcoming space to seek help.

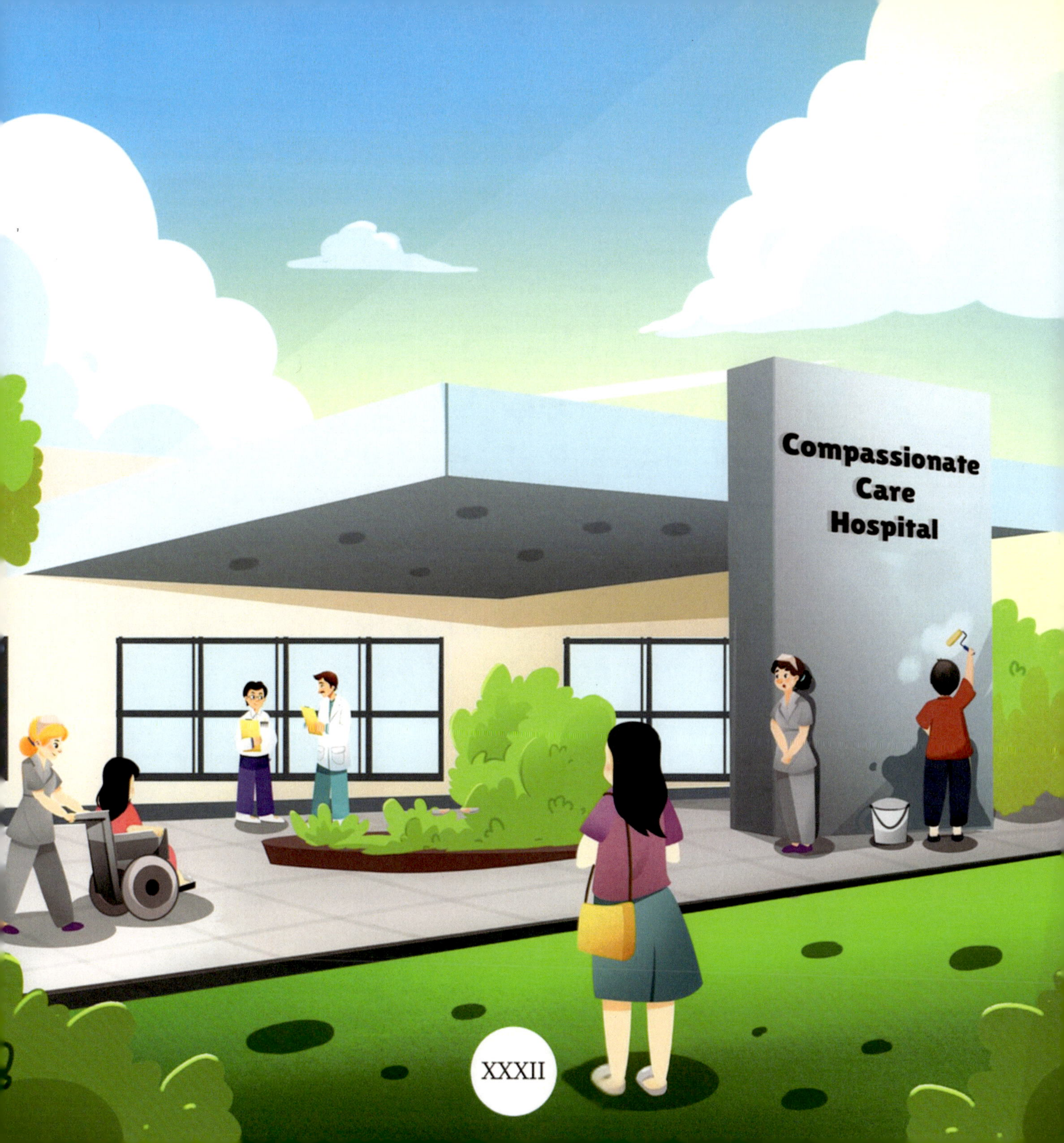
Compassionate
Care
Hospital

Travis transformed a challenging situation into a positive outcome. Even amidst judgment and discouragement, he remained true to his calling and didn't let anyone hinder his purpose. Although there will always be skeptics, Travis knows that if he can change even one person's life, he has fulfilled God's work. For this reason, he will always be considered a hero, his influence has shape other mental patients and staff members to be better of self discipline and self love that results a better impact and the world of mankind.

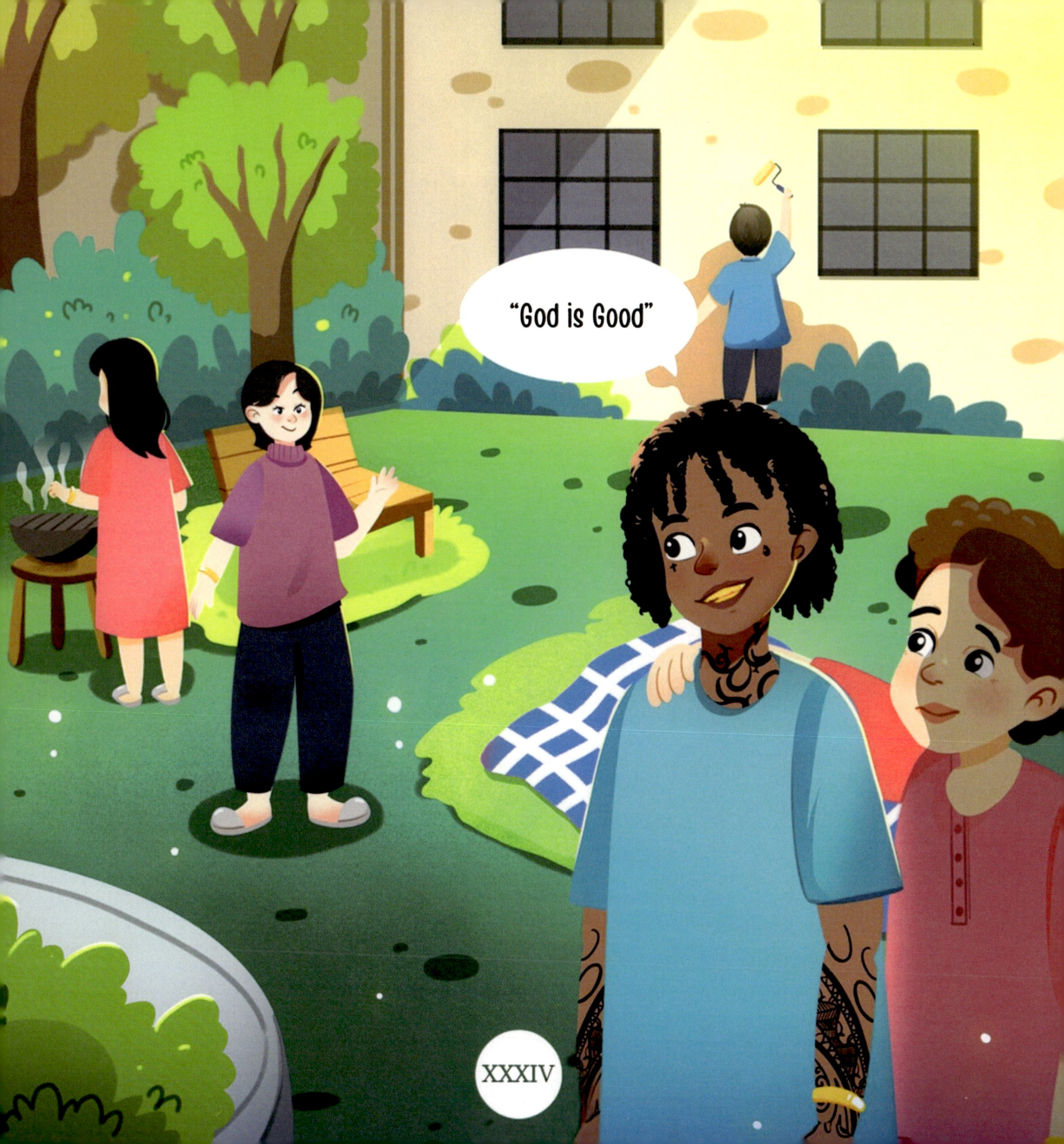
"God is Good"

Author's Ending Response

As this story draws to a close, remember that the path of healing and hope is never easy. It takes courage to stand firm when faced with doubt, strength to show kindness in a world too often marked by cruelty, and faith to carry a light when others question its source. The journey of the anointed healer teaches us that true transformation comes not from appearance or acceptance, but from a heart willing to serve despite the odds.

Now, as you close this book, I leave you with one final question—one that challenges us all to look within:

"Could you endure the weight of doubt, the sting of pain, and the sting of judgment-and still choose compassion over comfort, obedience over fear, and the will of God over your own self-preservation?"

Author's Letter

"Mental awareness is something I take very seriously. Growing up in a two-parent household, I was always taught to understand that everyone has a story to tell; not everyone is delusional. I learned that every emotional action has a backstory; some individuals really just want love and crying out for help. Most people diagnosed with a mental disorder have gone through something in life, and often, no one was there to comfort them or fill the void of love and encouragement. As a society, we should all play our part and embody the leadership qualities that reside within us. There are many different cultures, religions, and nationalities around the world, but we can all agree on what is right and what is wrong—an understanding shared by each individual. If we know better, we will do better. Mental illness often comes from rejection, trauma, and abuse across various contexts, which can lead to depression that sometimes pushes the human mind to a place of no return. Some may disagree with my opinion, but if we take the time to show concern, have an ear to hear, and protect one another, the world would be a much better place. Mental illness wouldn't be at an all-time high. Love is free; let's not cost each other the pain and suffering. God bless you all."

Sincerely,

Cameron Rod Mitchell Jr

www.ingramcontent.com/pod-product-compliance
Lightning Source LLC
LaVergne TN
LVRC080248220926
848482LV00042B/352

* 9 7 9 8 3 4 9 5 7 4 4 1 2 *